Mana Sciences

EMPOWER
ME
FREE
YOGA

Dedicated to advancing the Hawaiian art of personal empowerment for the body, mind & spirit.

EMPOWER ME FREE YOGA

Empower Your Yoga Practice with Hawaiian-Style Mana!

Keti Kamalani & Michelle Shine, Ph.D.

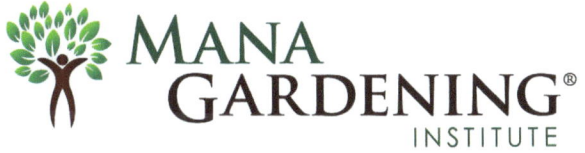

MANA
GARDENING®
INSTITUTE

What is Mana Sciences^{TM} Hawaiian-Style Yoga?

Ancient Hawaiians discovered the secrets of empowerment from within. Ancient yoga gurus unlocked the power of human transformation. Mana Sciences Yoga blends the two together to physically empower and transform your life. Discover more from every yoga pose and access your own inner power through our Hawaiian-style Suvasana.

Mana Sciences uses ancient Hawaiian methods of going within to empower your body, mind and soul. Mana Sciences Yoga utilizes our unique, self-guided *on-the-go* meditation to feel energized, or relaxed, as wanted or needed, anytime, anywhere. Discover the skills you were born with and live a better life! Learn how to empower yourself and your yoga practice with Hawaiian-style *Mana*!

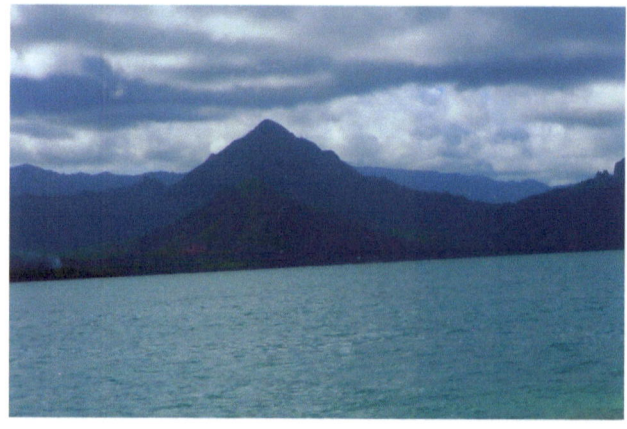

Mana Sciences, aligned with Hatha yoga principals, presents our *Empower Me Free* practice to compliment every style of yoga. This book is a reference guide for all yoga enthusiasts who want to deepen their practice with Hawaiian tools of empowerment.

Yoga instructors can become certified in Mana Sciences Yoga. Our program teaches *Mana Gardening* personal empowerment techniques adapted to the practice of yoga. Training offers in-depth studies in the three corners of the Mana Sciences pyramid through: *Empower Me Free Yoga*, *No Go Yoga*, and *On-The-Go Meditation*.

What Do You Mean by *EMPOWER ME FREE?*

Learn our self-guided, empowering, real-life skills to free yourself from the addiction of negative energy and let happiness become your way of life. If you would like a better understanding of these principals, visit our website or check out our book, *Mana Gardening, Empower Yourself & Live a Better Life.* You can find out more about us at www.managardening.com

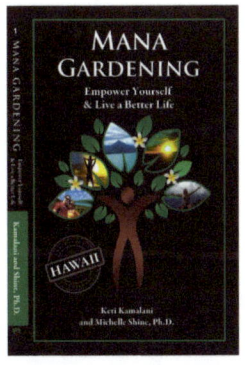

Empower Me Free Yoga takes you through one of our yoga flows using Hawaiian and *Mana Gardening* terms and techniques. This flow covers the following five principals of *Mana Gardening*:

1. Add valuable Hawaiian principals to the start of your everyday yoga practice.

2. Let go of stress, fear and worry by pulling negative energy out of your body and releasing it through simple poses.

3. Create a force field of protective energy with a pattern of poses that guard you from negative influences.

4. Access your inner paradise to relax and rejuvenate by moving inward through *on-the-go* meditation while moving through sun salutations and restorative poses.

5. Deepen your Suvasana as you discover your inner *Mana* to bring healthy energy back to your day-to-day life.

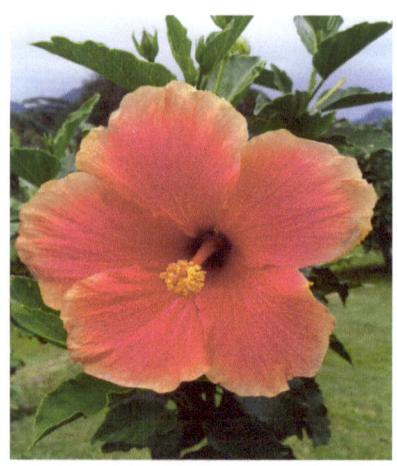

Pohaku Naholoholo

Before we get started with our *Empower Me Free Yoga* flow, you will need to create a set of Hawaiian traveling stones to be used in our unique Suvasana. Every participant must have two stones, so instructors will need to make a larger number of stones. If you are practicing on your own, you will still need to create your own Hawaiian-style traveling stones which we call **Pohaku Naholoholo**.

Instructors will need a large bowl filled with these stones. Practicing on your own will require at least one stone with each design. The following pages guide you in creating your own stones and shares with you some Hawaiian words and concepts. In Mana Sciences Yoga you become your own guru, however that does not replace the importance of learning yoga with the guidance of certified instructor.

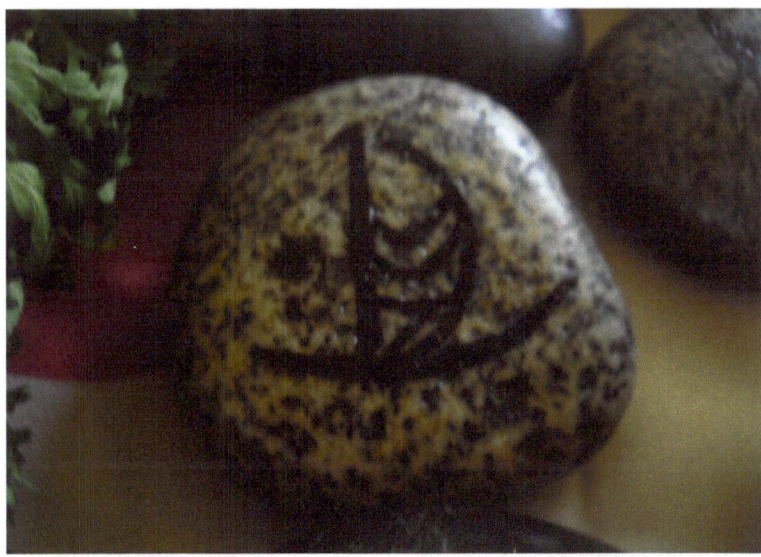

Mana

Hawaiians believe that everything has a positive spiritual strength or **Mana** and the ability to absorb forthright energy. We use stones to teach you how this works, however, in Hawaii it is **Kapu,** or forbidden, to take stones from where they live. Use stones like river rock as traveling has been part of their life cycle. We buy them from the hardware store and call them Pohaku Naholoholo, meaning stones that have followed the stars.

Create your own Pohaku Naholoholo with smooth stones, a sharpie, coconut oil and happy music. Turn the music on, rinse the stones in water and dry them off. Enjoy the music as all the powerful *Mana* passes through your hands.

With the sharpie draw symbols from the next pages onto the stones. Create a variety of stones. Feel the energy of the water, the strength of the stones, the healing of the coconut oil, and the pride of your good work. Have fun and don't worry for the perfection of your art.

When finished, massage the stones by hand with coconut oil and say, "Mahalo, nui loa" to thank them for their gift to you. We will use these stones in **Suvasana.** When you begin your yoga practice select two stones and place them just off your mat. For now, when you finish making all of your stones just set them aside for later, preferably in a wooden bowl.

Historical Hawaiian Images

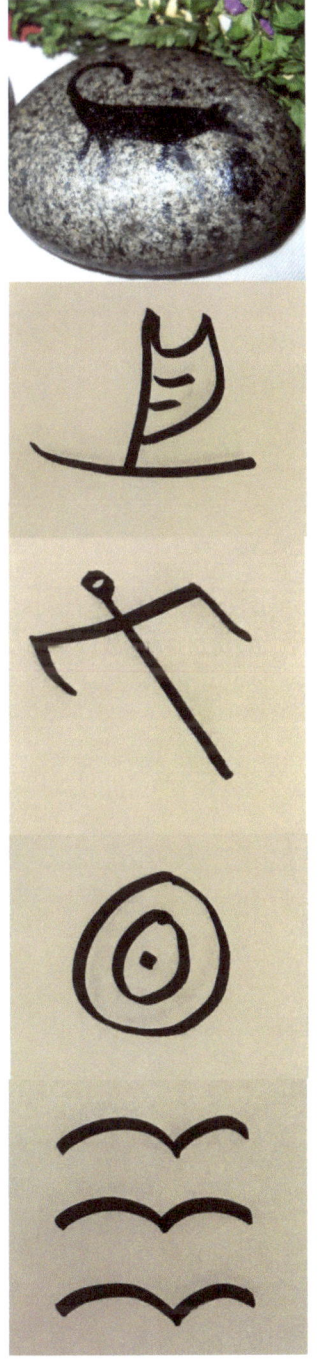

Lio = Dog
Poi Dog
Faithful
Friend

Travel
Freedom
Adventure

Bird
Freedom

Third Eye
Insight
Understanding

Flock
Journey
Trust

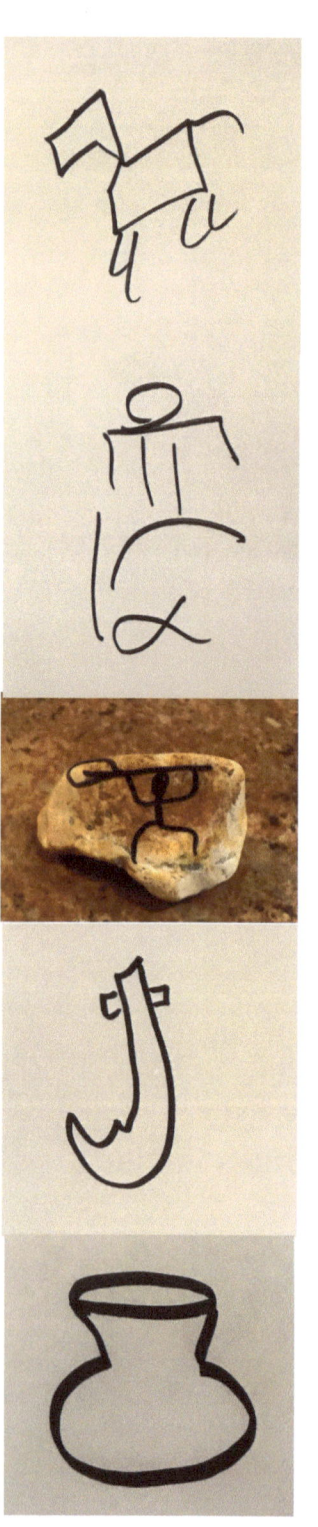

Ilio = Horse
Freedom
Spirit
Independent

Fisherman
Provider
Stability
Faithful

Splintered Paddle
Justice granted

Fishing hook
Faith
Stability
Ability to succeed

Ipu
Music
Happiness
Dance

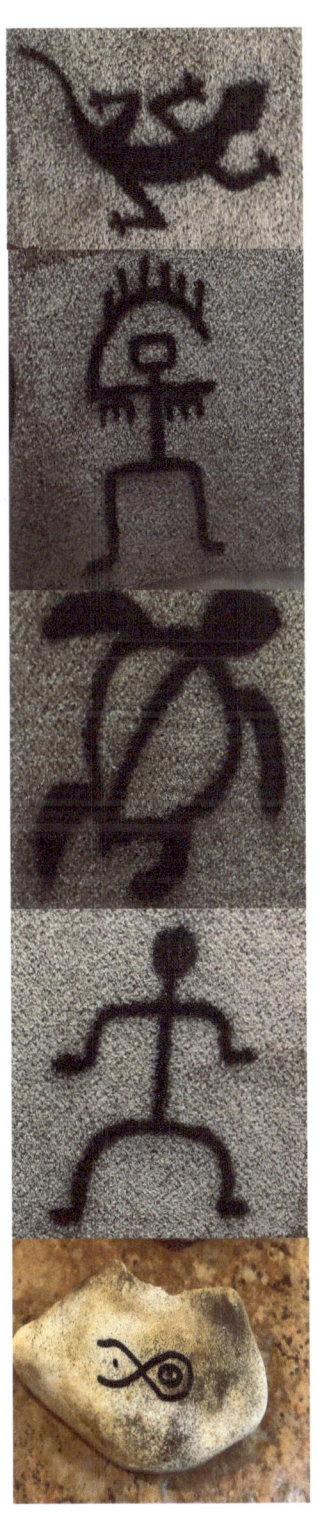

Gecko
Resilience
Agility
Tenacity

Ali'i = Royalty
Chief
Wisdom
Insight

Honu = Turtle
Wise
Steadfast
Adventurous

Kane = Man
Strength
Capable

Healing
Navigation
Spiritual

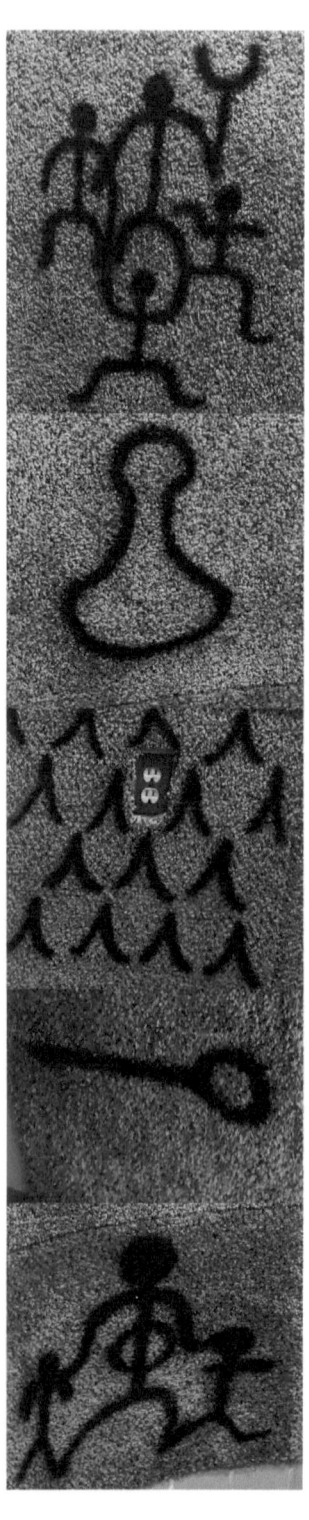

Leadership
Strength
Guidance
Teacher

Poi Pounder
Nourish
Provide

Mountains
Challenges
Perseverance
Strength

Paddle
Navigation
Law

Wahine = Woman
Secure
Nurture

The images have multiple positive meanings which may not be listed. They may also have their own personal significance to you. We suggest you consider your own thoughts on each image. Store the stones in a wood or clay bowl.

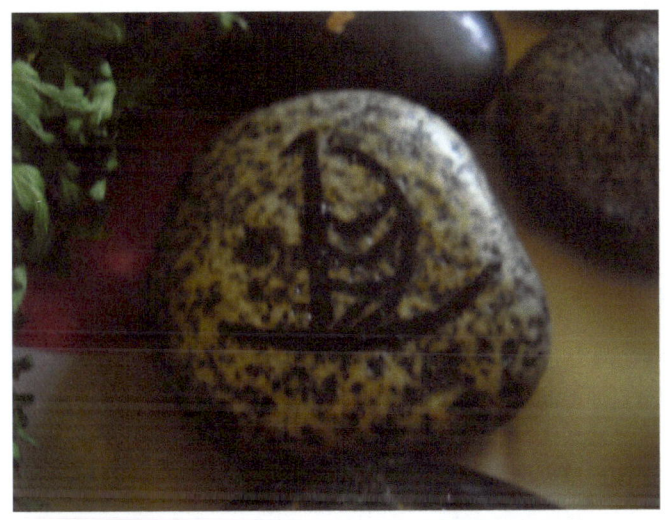

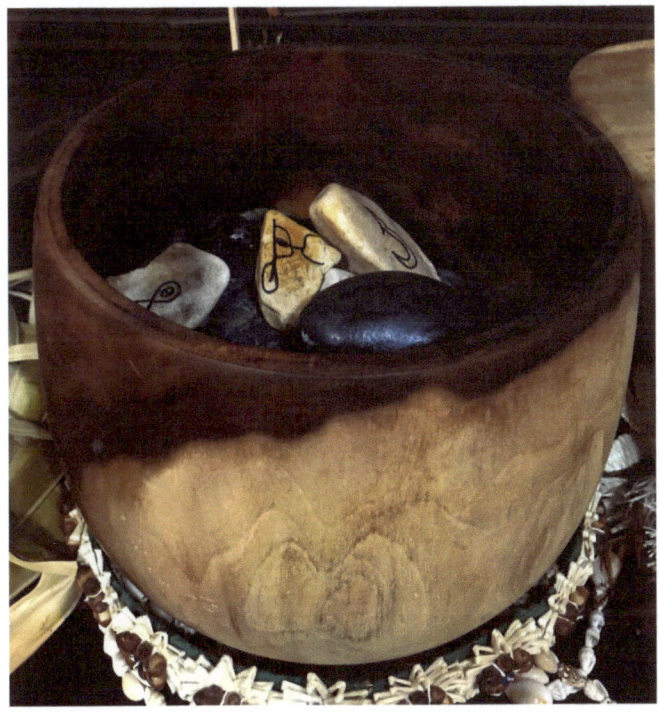

Hawaiian Words & Concepts

We have already shared the terms of *Mana* for spiritual energy and empowerment, Kapu for forbidden, Pohaku for stone, and Nahololo for following the stars. When we ask you to breathe, we will use the term **Ha.** Ha means the breath of life and it is so much more than breathing. Yoga guides us to focus on our breathing, drawing us to inhale deeply feeding the body and mind. Ancient Hawaiians valued the exhale, the Ha, as a powerful tool for healing. We will remind you often to inhale and exhale deeply, to empower your body and mind with nourishment and healing.

The Hawaiian culture teaches the practice of **Hoʻoponopono,** which means to make things right. Whenever you have a falling out with another person, no matter whose fault it was, putting an effort in to making things right can transform your life in a positive way. Yoga teaches us ways to transform ourselves for a life filled with energy, health and resiliency. To benefit from Mana Sciences Yoga, you must practice Hoʻoponopono. The Hawaiian practice requires that you work directly with the other person, but often that may not be possible. We suggest you read our original book *Mana Gardening, Empower Yourself and Live & Better Life,* to discover how you can easily make things right from within. With our techniques, you do not have to work with anyone else, it only takes you.

No trip to Hawaii is complete without a fresh flower **Lei** or hearing the term **Aloha**, but few understand their meanings. The Lei is the circle of life and represents the non-verbal spirit of Aloha. It symbolizes hope, joy, and love. Aloha can mean many beautiful things: hello, farewell, respect, honor, and celebration. When said, there is love in the present moment. When you see a Lei or hear the word, "Aloha," embrace the great love of that moment in time.

Mahalo means thank you. We prefer **Mahalo nui loa** which means a heartfelt and sincere thank you or you're welcome. We invite you to add Hawaiian words to your yoga practice. Lastly, Hawaiians see *Mana* as an empowering inner force of life and nature, so open your eyes not just to the beauty around you, but within you too!

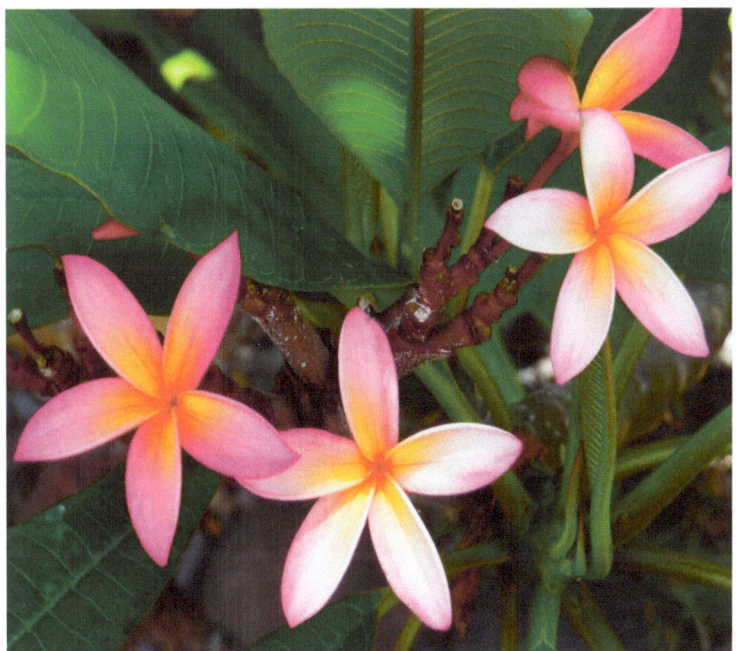

The Beauty of Yoga

Our yoga practice embraces the elegance of **Fluidity** and the importance of **Ahimsa**. Fluidity is that free-flowing movement when rising up, standing, walking, running or even resting. We were fluid as children, thriving in our growth and feeling capable in trying new things. Feeling fluid should be smooth and easy, like a child reaching for the sky!

Ahimsa is a devotion to avoid harming ourselves and others. Mana Sciences Yoga was influenced by the yoga teachings of Murti Hower and his wife Larina Hawkins-Hower. They teach Ahimsa through proper posture and alignment to protect our bodies from unnecessary pain and impingements. We ask you to respect the beauty of yoga by placing Fluidity and Ahimsa at the center of your yoga practice.

Our goal is to empower you through one of our unique yoga flows. This book was designed to compliment your yoga practice and not as a comprehensive manual. To learn yoga we suggest that you work with a Registered Yoga Teacher (RYT). As you practice, pay attention to how you move in each pose and focus inward on yourself. Breath deeply pairing your movements with an inhale or an exhale.

Before you roll out your mat to practice yoga, always run a posture pre-check. Make sure you have good posture. You may need to put some effort into correcting your posture. With the use of cell phones and computers our bodies no longer understand what good posture really means. Bad posture has become so profound that our scapula's tend to wing out even when we sleep.

To check your posture, stand up straight with the top half of your back flat against a wall. Your shoulders should not touch the wall. There should be a natural curve of the spine creating a space at the lower part of your back. Only the upper back and your rear end should touch the wall. Your head, neck, shoulders, legs, hips and feet should be aligned straight.

This is good posture and it is vital to a long, healthy life. In everything you do, strive for good posture. Check yourself often and break the bad habit of slouching with rolled shoulders and a curved spine. Learn to hold your head up with pride and self-respect.

Changing Our Perspective

Let's begin our yoga flow by embracing the Hawaiian culture. Take two stones and set them by your mat. Say, "Aloha," out loud and come into **Tadasana** or **Mountain** pose. Check your posture. Breathe in deeply, hold your breath slightly and the exhale slowly saying, "Ha." This helps to heal us and everything around us.

Now we are ready to let go of the negative energy within us. Imagine all your hardships, struggles, and sorrows bubbling up and traveling to your shoulders, flowing down your arms and into your hands. See the worries slipping out of your mind, leaving your head and neck and flowing to your hands. Feel your hands become heavy.

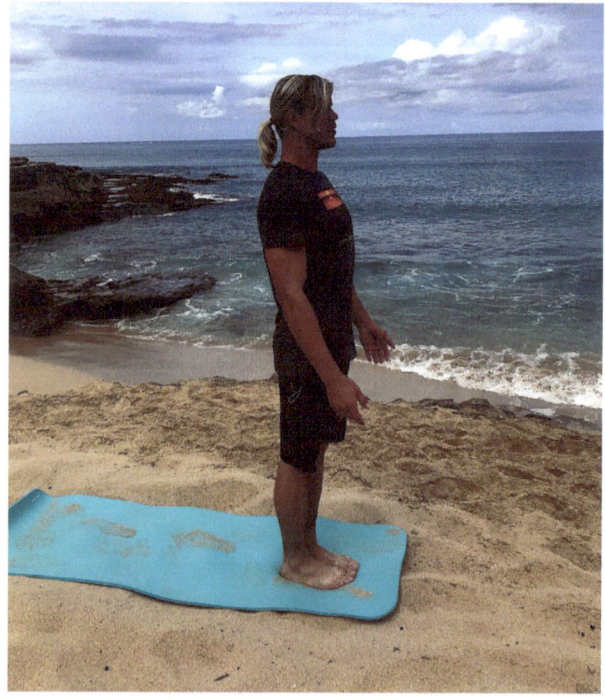

Move into **Urdhva Hastasana,** also known as **Volcano** pose. Exhale slowly saying, "Ha," and reach upward with both hands. Imagine all of the hurt, pain, anger and disappointment from life, flowing out from your hands. Open your hands and let all your struggles go. See and feel the stress leaving your body and freeing your mind. *Mana Gardening* teaches us that the only thing we have the power to change is our perspective. Reach upward and believe that you have let go of the hurt and the worries. You are ready to see your life in a positive light and create the changes you want or need.

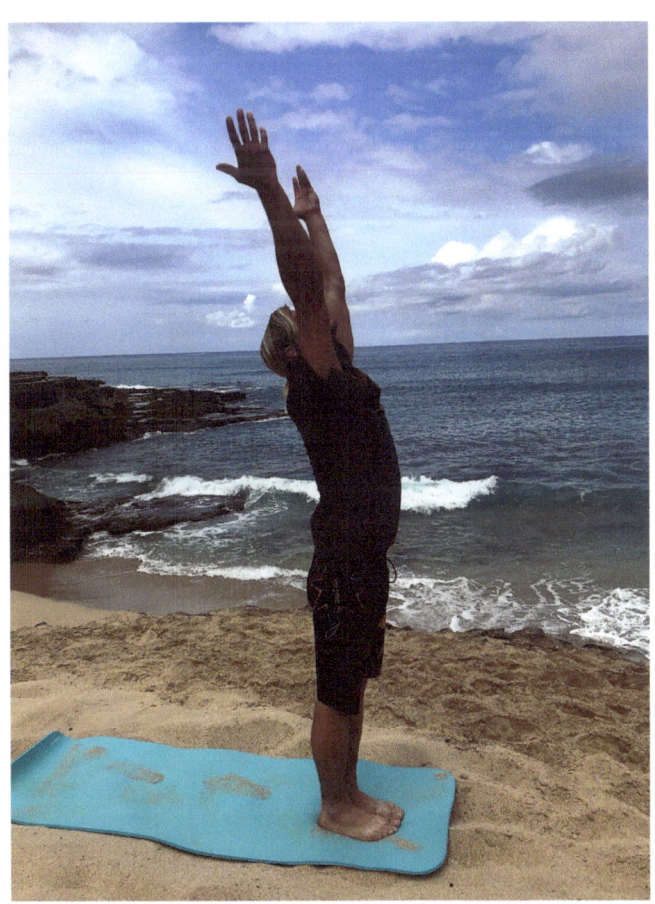

Bend forward into a **Standing Forward Bend** or **Uttanasana**. Take a bow and honor the power of the universe. Free of negative energy, you now have space to refill yourself with great *Mana*. Feel yourself breathe. In each pose we move with intent. We take our time. We hold the pose breathing in and out deeply.

Remember to focus on Fluidity and Ahimsa. Bend only as much as it feels comfortable. When you exhale, pull your chest inward towards your knees and ask that all that is great and forthright reside within you. Breathe the Ha of life, and feel it within you.

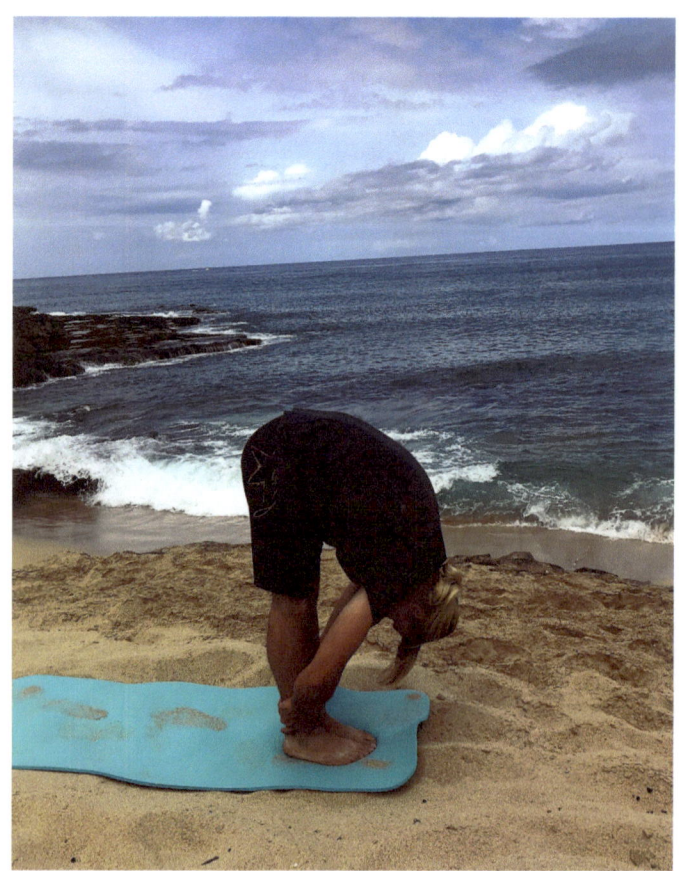

The Protective Energy

Creating a force field of protective energy requires following through several poses as we visualize an energy wall rising up around us. Starting with the right foot back, we circle the mat turning to the right with each new pose. When finished, we will repeat the entire force field starting with the left foot back and turning to your left.

Begin with **Virabhadrasana I, or Warrior I**. Feel the strength from within you and imagine a shield of energy around you. With each pose, feel a wall of energy with your hands and feet. Claim this as your space to become empowered, happy and strong. Let the wind blow as it will. You arc frcc from negative energy.

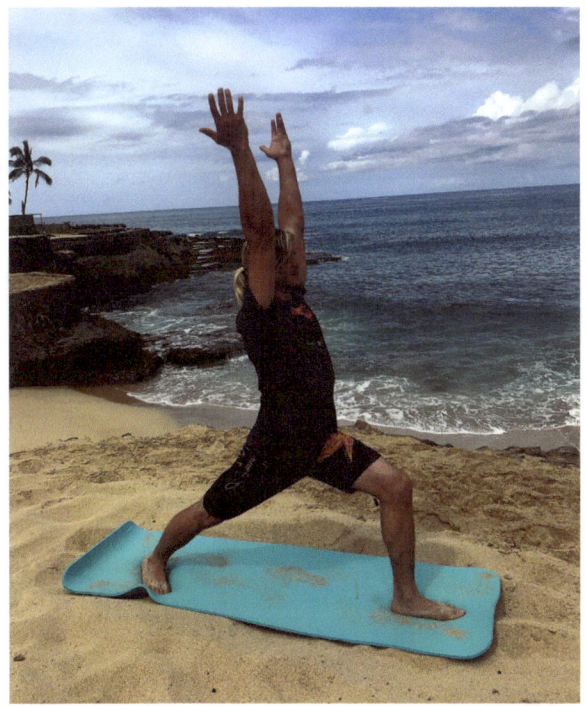

Pivot on your right foot and move into **Warrior II** or **Virabhadrasana II.** This is your space and you have a right to be here. Breathe deeply and slowly. Building this wall of energy will take some time and effort. See the force field rising up in front of you. Feel it rising up behind you. Your fingers can touch it, your feet are standing on it.

Move slowly and remember that all of the negative energy has left you. There is a new space within you to fill with powerful *Mana*. Like the warrior, hold your head high with pride. Check your posture, make sure both scapula's are flat and not winging out stressing your head and neck. Let the back arm pull you into proper posture and alignment.

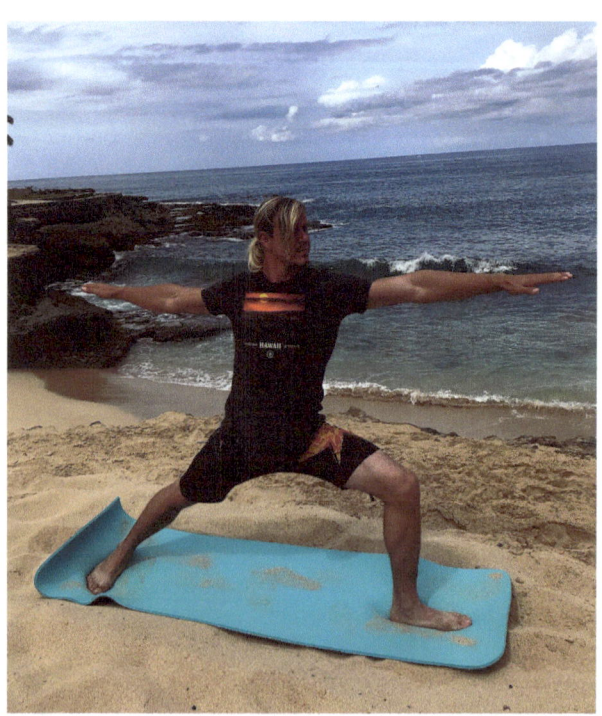

Pivot your left foot parallel with the right foot. Move into **Wide-Legged Standing Forward Bend, Prasarita Padottanasana.** Step out wide. There are many variations of this pose, from hands to the floor, hands on your ankles, or using a block to bring your back straight and support the torso.

Visualize the force field underneath you as it surrounds you side to side, back to front, and top to bottom. You are building a thick wall of powerful energy that will surround you on all sides and deflect negative energy.

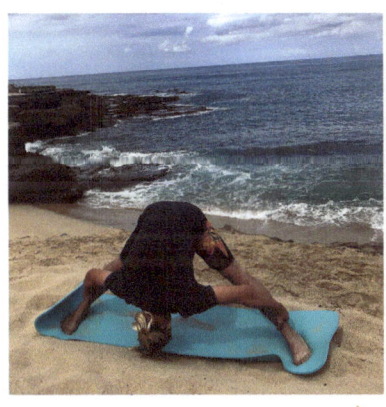 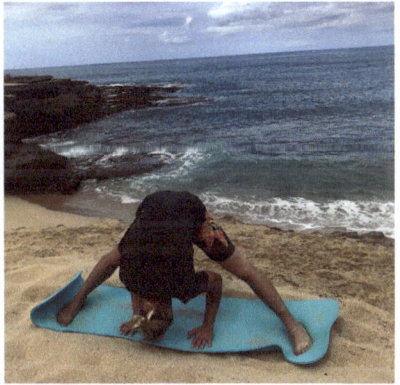

Imagine that your feet are standing on this wall of energy, and your head and hands are resting on it as it rises up around you. With the head lower than the heart, this pose is a mild inversion known for it is calming qualities.

Stabilize the legs to protect your lower back but do not lock the knees. To come back up, move your hands onto your hips, bend the knees slightly, and come up slowly.

Turn right with your arms up, pivot your right foot until it is pointed to the back and move into **Virabhadrasana II,** or **Warrior II.** This time you are facing the back of the mat. You are now half way through the first circle moving right.

In Warrior II, be sure that you can see your big toe, but not your smaller toes. Use your back arm to pull your torso straight aligning your back and spine. Are you breathing? Don't forget to breathe. Exhale and inhale fully. Check your posture. Align your head with your neck.

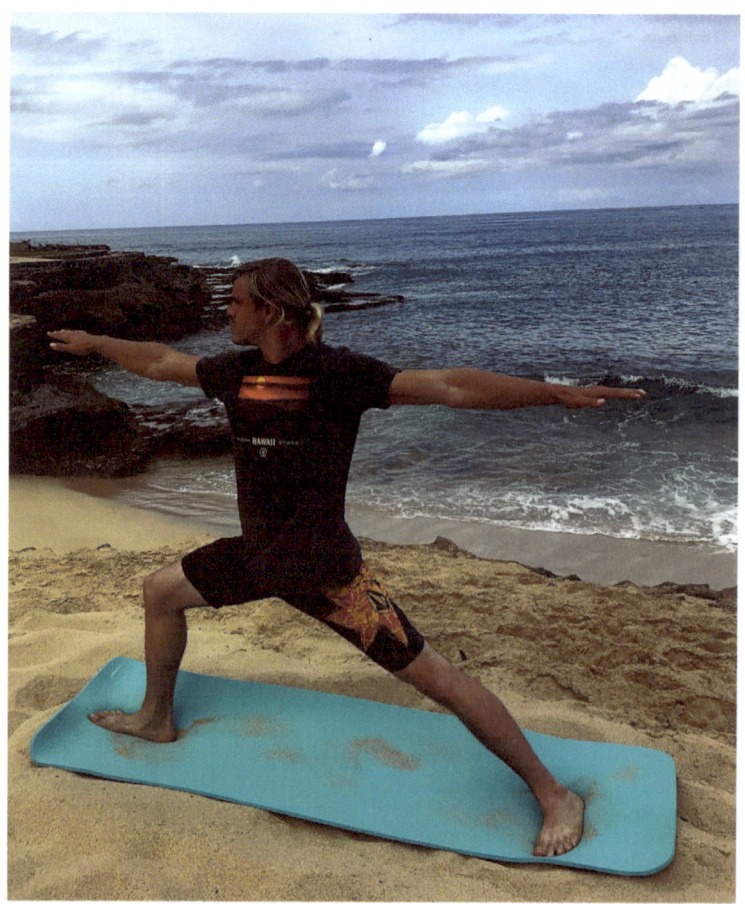

Pivot your left foot and turn your body towards the right. You will now be facing the opposite direction of where you started building your energy force field. Plant both feet down firmly. Spread your full weight evenly out to all sides of your feet. Lift up your toes, spread them out wide and bring them all down as anchors to support your legs. Pushing downward on both feet, stretch your arms up as you move into **Virabhadrasana I** or **Warrior I.** This pose has great *Mana*. Breathe deeply in and out feeling empowered from within.

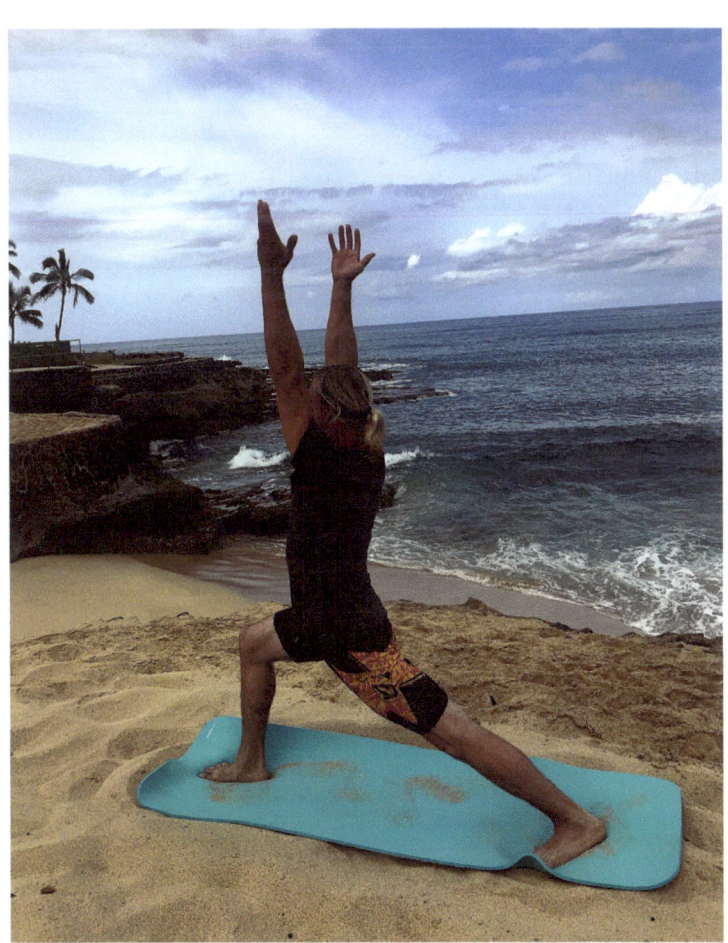

Place your weight onto the right foot. Use your entire foot–the heel, the pad of your foot, and the toes–to stabilize your right leg. Lean forward with both hands out, coming up onto your right foot and into **Warrior III** or **Virabhadrasana III.** Push out the force field wall to make more space in your inner circle. Feel the wall becoming thicker and stronger as it resists you.

This inner circle is yours and is surrounded by a lifetime force field to guard you from negative energy. Feel your own positive energy safe within its thick, powerful walls. Lift the back leg high to remain balanced. Focusing on the back leg rising upward and the full exhale of the Ha takes you deeper into each pose and helps you retain your balance. When you come out of this pose, plant both feet side-by-side, say, "Mahalo nui loa," and feel thankful.

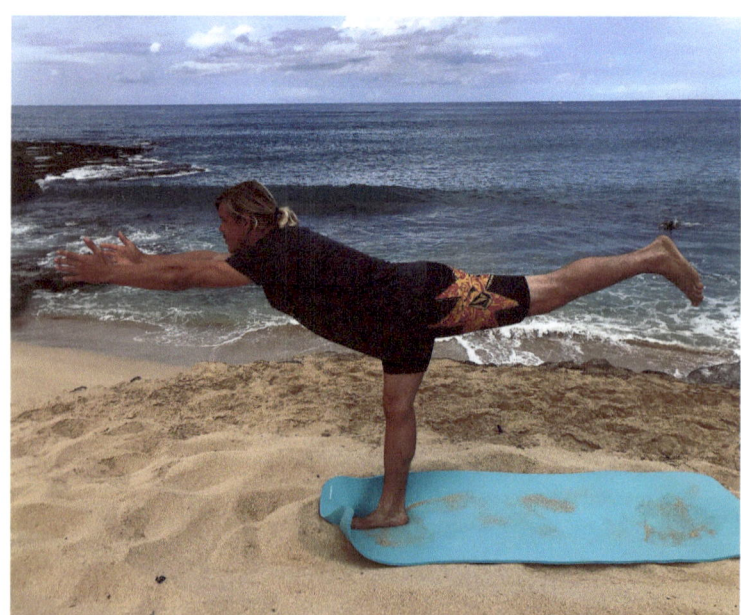

Step back with your right foot. Plant both feet down firmly. Is your full weight evenly spread out to all sides of your feet? Did you lift up your toes, and spread them out wide to anchor your stand? Move smoothly into **Warrior I** or **Virabhadrasana I.** Creating the force field should feel repetitive as we work to strengthen all sides. Moving from pose to pose, strive for Fluidity and Ahimsa.

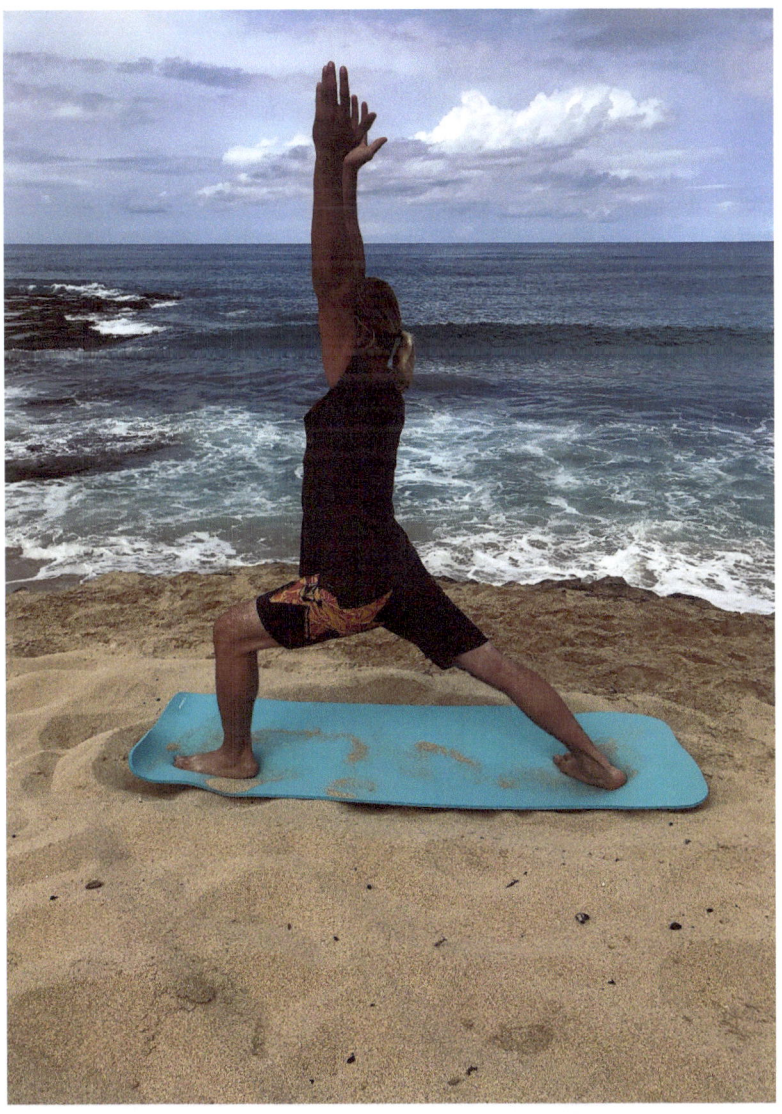

Pivot your right foot and float both arms out into **Warrior II, Virabhadrasana II.** Now that you are getting used to the sequence, you can focus on safely flowing in and out of each pose. Fluidity, firm footing and good posture should all begin to feel more and more natural.

The purpose of this part of our flow is to protect our positive new perspective by creating a force field to shield us from negative energy that safeguards us from every direction. Turn the left foot to the right so that both feet are parallel to one another. Step out wider and float your arms down into **Prasarita Padottanasana,** or **Wide-Legged Standing Forward Bend**.

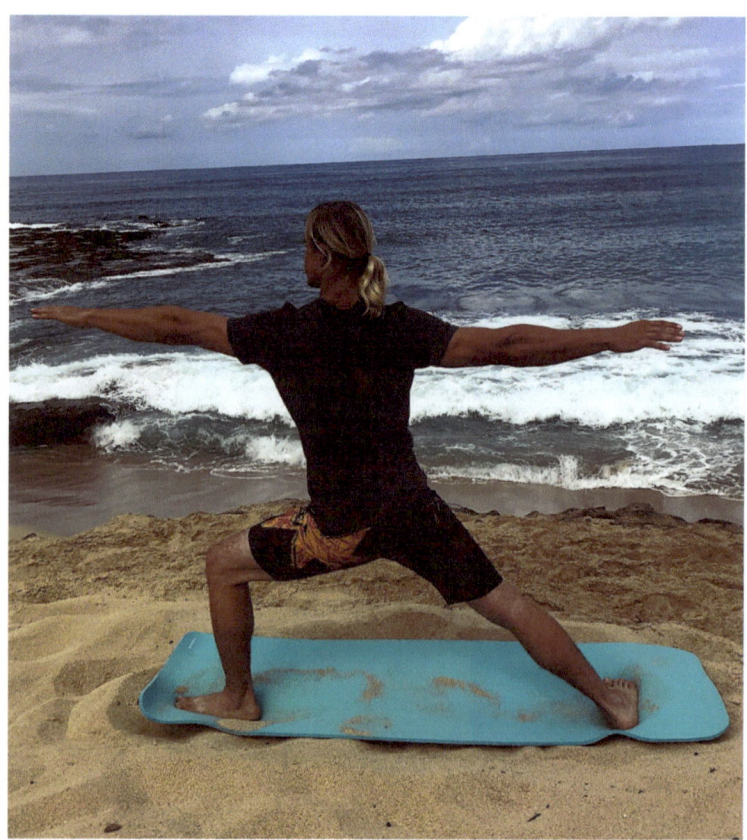

Now facing the other side, remember that you can experiment with different variations, perhaps moving your hands from your ankles to the floor in front of you for more support. Relax your face, head, neck and shoulders. Let your head hang weightlessly. As you breathe in allow your chest to fill with air and rise out away from your legs. On the exhale let your chest sink closer to your legs and body.

If your weight is on your hands, bend your elbows. A wider stance will keep your back straight. Scan yourself for any impingements and adjust yourself so that this pose is enjoyable. If you still feel uncomfortable, place your hands on a block or chair to support your shoulders and lower back. When you come out of this pose, bring your feet closer together and place your hands on your hips rising back up.

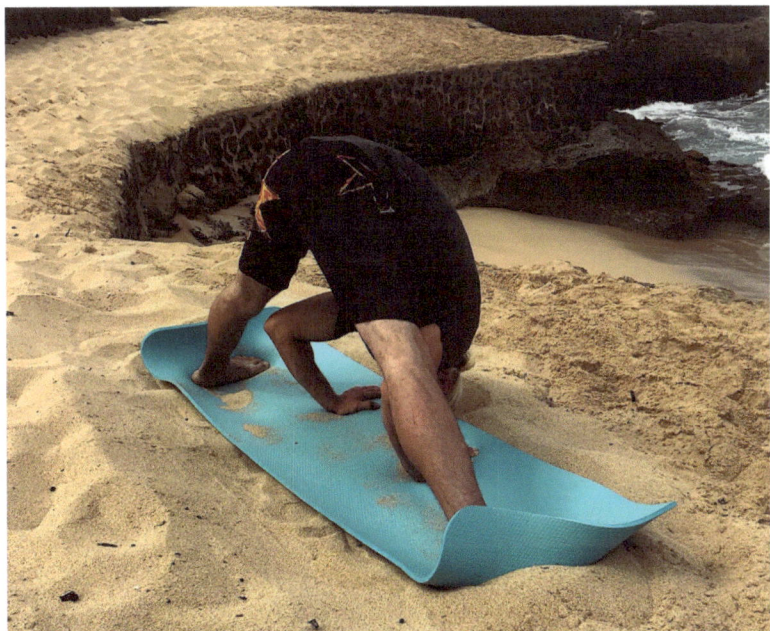

The right-sided full circle is almost done. Keep turning right pivoting your right foot until it is pointed to the front of your mat where we first began. Glide back into **Virabhadrasana II,** or **Warrior II**. We have now completed our first circle and built a force field . Breathe the Ha.

Feel empowered as the force field surrounds you. Gaze down your arms, across your hands and over your fingertips looking at the force field in front of you. Close your eyes and try to feel it behind you, just beyond you.

Embrace the positive energy within the circle. You are safe from the negative influences that bombard us from every direction. Negativity is addictive, it is everywhere. Empowered, you are free from negativity. Bathe yourself in the positive energy.

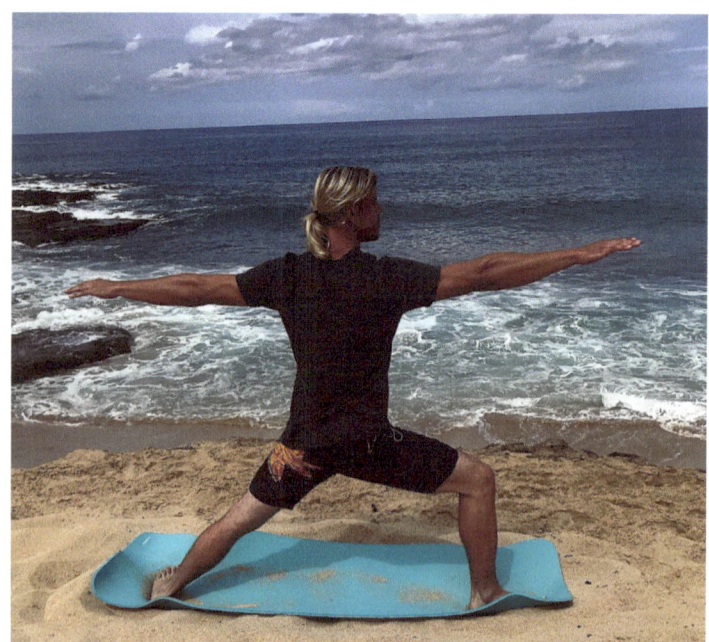

Rotate both feet towards the front of your mat. You are back where you first started. Once again plant both feet down firmly, spread out your toes and anchor your right foot moving into **Warrior I** or **Virabhadrasana I.**

Self-adjust the slight backwards curve of the spine so it feels good. Reach for the sky with both hands. Extend your arms upward and feel it lengthen your spine. Keep your back leg up and do not let your hips or pelvis sink lower.

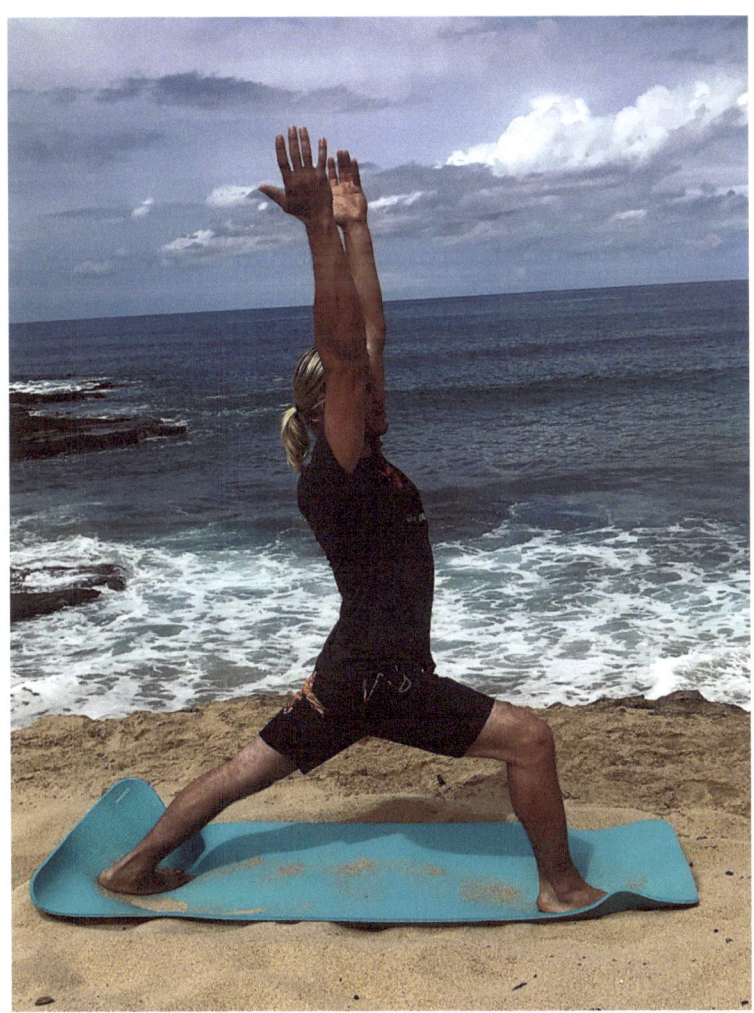

Check your right foot to ensure your toes are well-anchored and your weight is evenly distributed to your right foot. Float forward into **Warrior III,** or **Virabhadrasana III.** Push out against the force field with your hands to feel its resistance and the sheer strength of the energy that now surrounds you.

Bring your back leg up high to keep your balance and hold this pose as long as you can. You made it through the full right circle. Feel proud as you bring your left leg back down and come into **Mountain** pose.

Think about the words, "Aloha" and "Mahalo," with love and appreciation for the strength of your body. Try saying "Aloha," out loud and exhale deeply rewarding yourself with the breath of life.

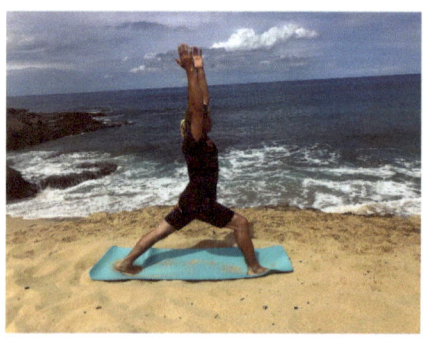 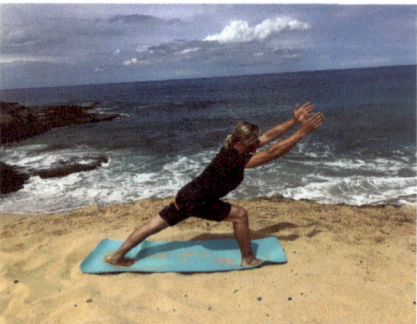

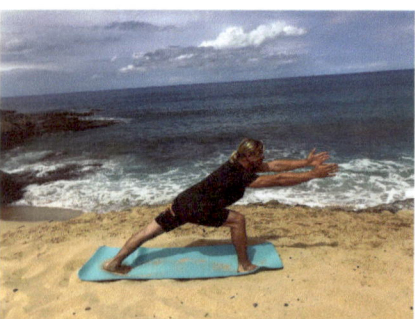 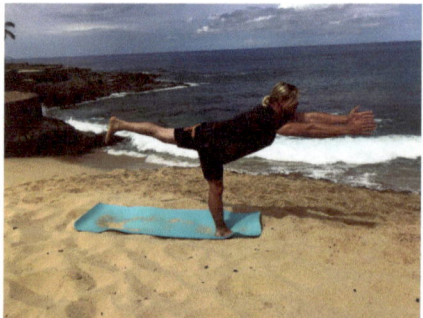

The Power of Circles

You must always circle both sides. In circling the left side, remain quiet and speak very little. The circle is a powerful life force like a beautiful Lei surrounding you. This protects your healthy perspective. Glide from pose to pose, focusing on strengthening the force field. As your thoughts wander, focus back to empowering yourself with strength and positive energy.

Begin the left circle at the front of your mat always moving left. Start in **Mountain** pose and slide your left foot back into **Warrior I**, then **Warrior II, Wide-Legged Standing Forward Bend**, back into **Warrior II, Warrior I** and **Warrior III**. Bring both feet side-by-side into **Mountain** pose facing the back of your mat. Keep turning left and move into **Warrior I, Warrior II, Wide-Legged Standing Forward Bend, Warrior II, Warrior I** and at last **Warrior III**. Stand up straight in **Mountain** pose, feeling empowered, grounded and centered in a powerful circle.

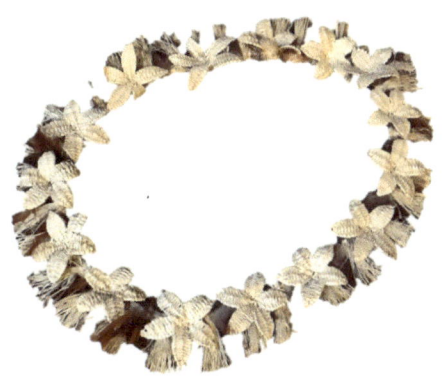

Moving Inward

Standing in **Mountain** pose, visualize the most peaceful or beautiful place you have ever seen, a place you dream of or love. Perhaps see yourself standing at the beach. Imagine the sounds that surround you. See this place as your garden, your paradise, your own personal heaven. Feel the warmth of the sun or the hint of a cool breeze. Breathe deeply with the Ha of life as you visualize your own private paradise here in your inner circle. Embrace the inner Aloha, the Mahalo nui loa of a thankful heart. Only positive energy is allowed here. Now the fun begins as you explore and journey inward. We will move through a sun salutation that you can modify however you prefer.

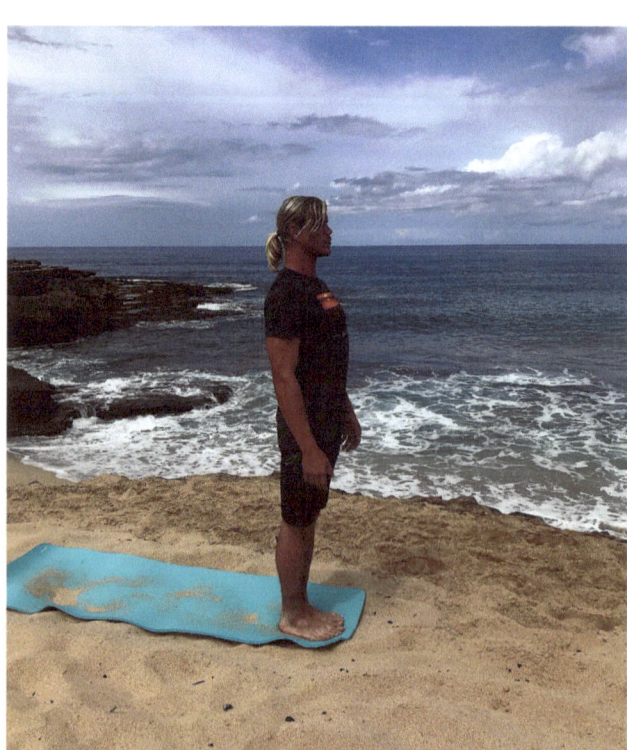

Reach both hands upward into **Volcano** pose holding on to that image of you in your beautiful paradise. Do not let the mind wander from this perfect place. At first you may need to close your eyes to see yourself in this place. We call this inner visualizing, *Mana Gardening*.

Open your eyes while still seeing yourself there in your inner garden. Enjoy the calm, peaceful feeling within you. Feel the positive energy of your force field on all sides. There is so much power around you and within you and yet this inner space seems endless. Bring both arms down slowly and move into a forward bend.

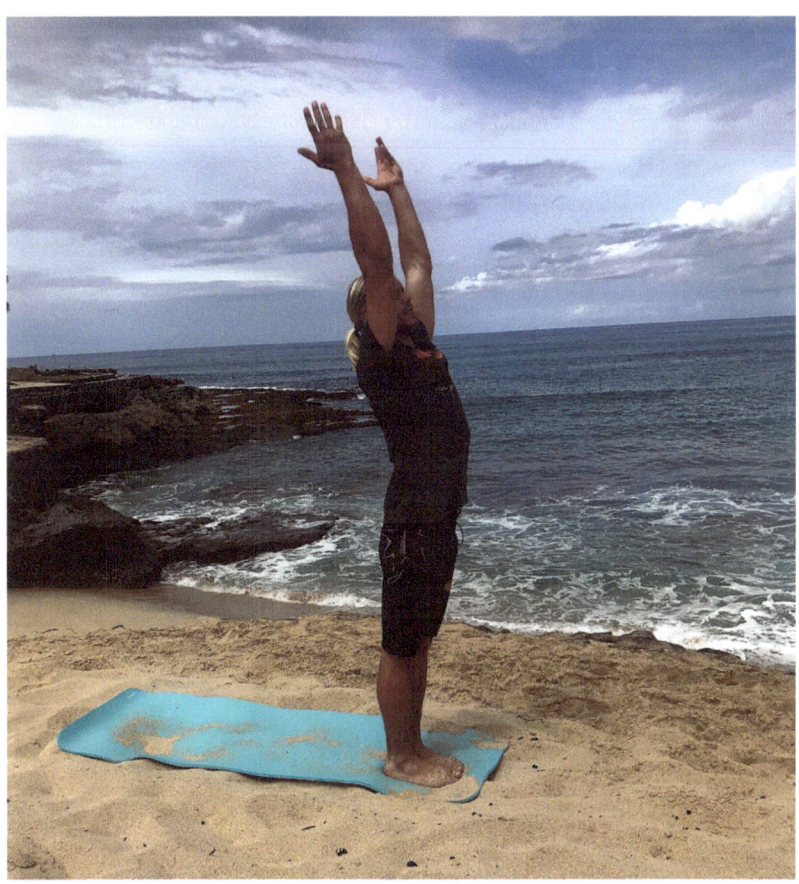

Try to flow freely from pose to pose. Lean into the **Forward Bend** or **Uttanasana** with your entire upper body suspended weightlessly. Breathe deeply and exhale with a Ha. Feel your body rise and relax with each and every breath. Take time to hold each pose for several full inhales and exhales.

Let the image of your inner garden, the beach or that peaceful, beautiful place soothe you. As you go through these next yoga movements the challenge is to keep returning your mind to this beautiful inner garden image with you there. When ready to come out of this pose, soften your legs by slightly bending your knees.

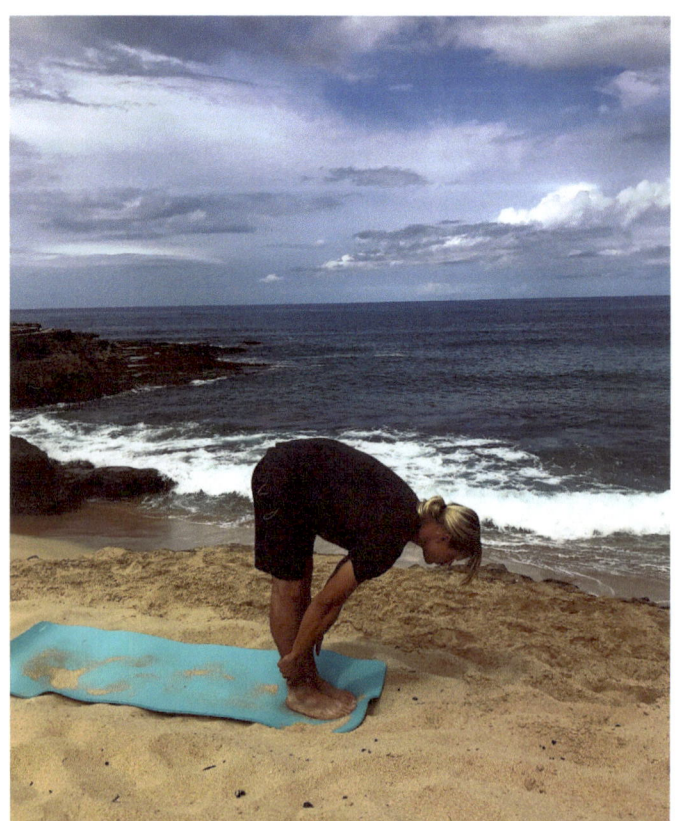

Extend both arms out in front of you to touch the ground. Nothing should hurt. You will stretch and work hard, but you should not be in pain. If your back needs support, use a block to bring the floor closer to your hands in this **Extended Forward Bend**.

Look upward holding the image of your inner garden in your mind and see yourself in that beautiful place. Feel your body relax each time you think of your garden. Seeing yourself there as you move through each pose is what we call *on-the-go* meditation. Like the Ha, it is healing.

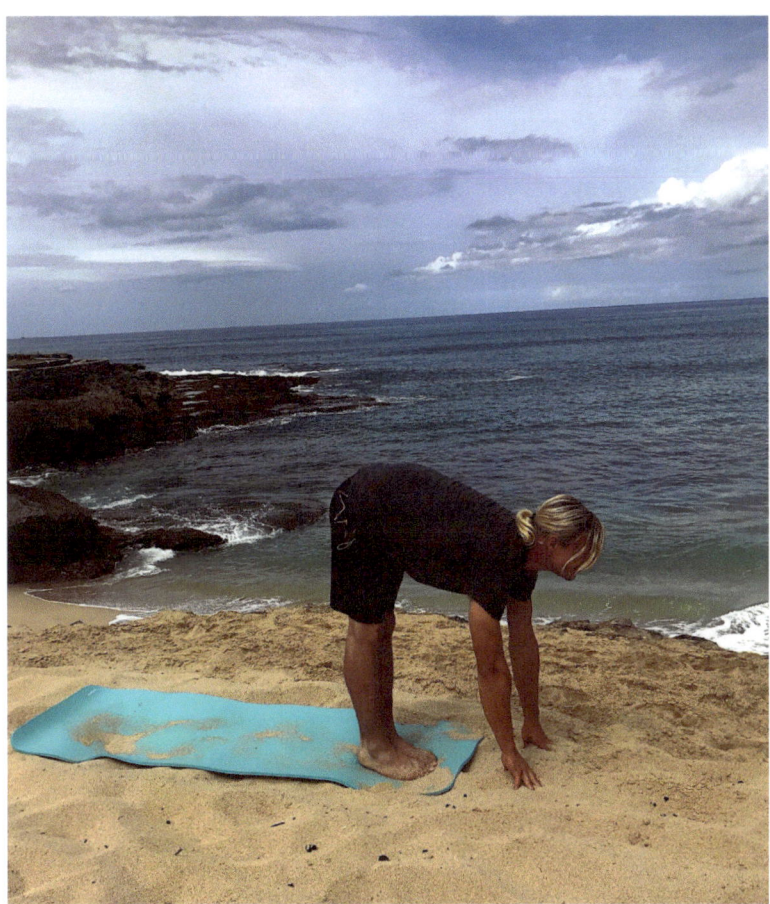

Place your hands beside your feet and move your right foot back into a runner's lunge. You may need to adjust your feet and hands. Look up and don't let the back leg drop down or the pelvis sink.

As you move from pose to pose see the positive energy around you strong and protective. Place yourself back into that beautiful inner garden and breathe deeply. Return your thoughts to your inner garden often.

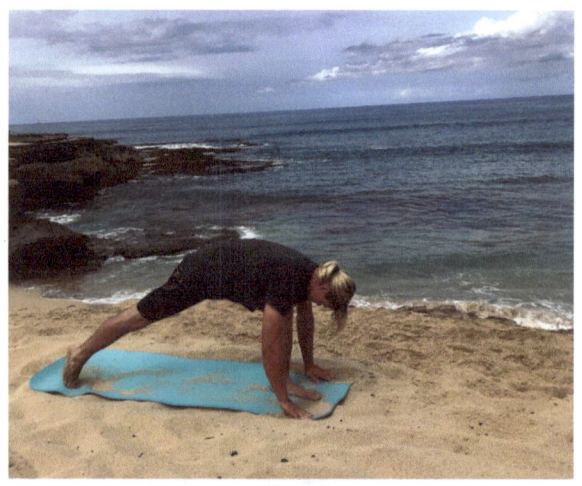

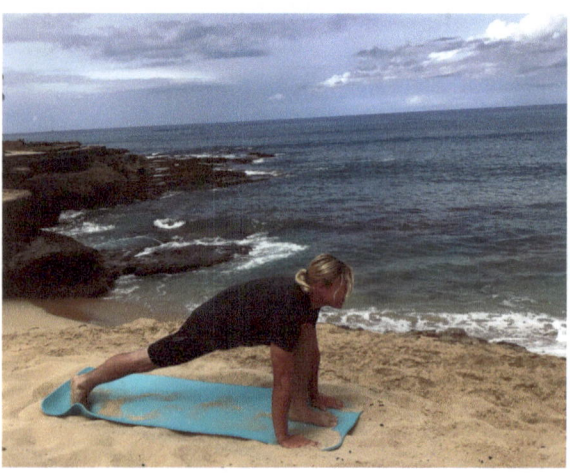

Move the left foot back and come into **Plank** pose. Tighten all of your muscles. Distribute the weight evenly to your arms and legs. Make sure your stomach, back and shoulders are sharing in the work. Bring your head up to ensure your neck and shoulders are not pinched.

Visualize your inner garden while looking straight ahead. Hold that image of yourself in the garden. Try dropping yourself back into your garden image every time you move your body. It takes practice to shift your body position and hold yourself in that beautiful place without losing your focus.

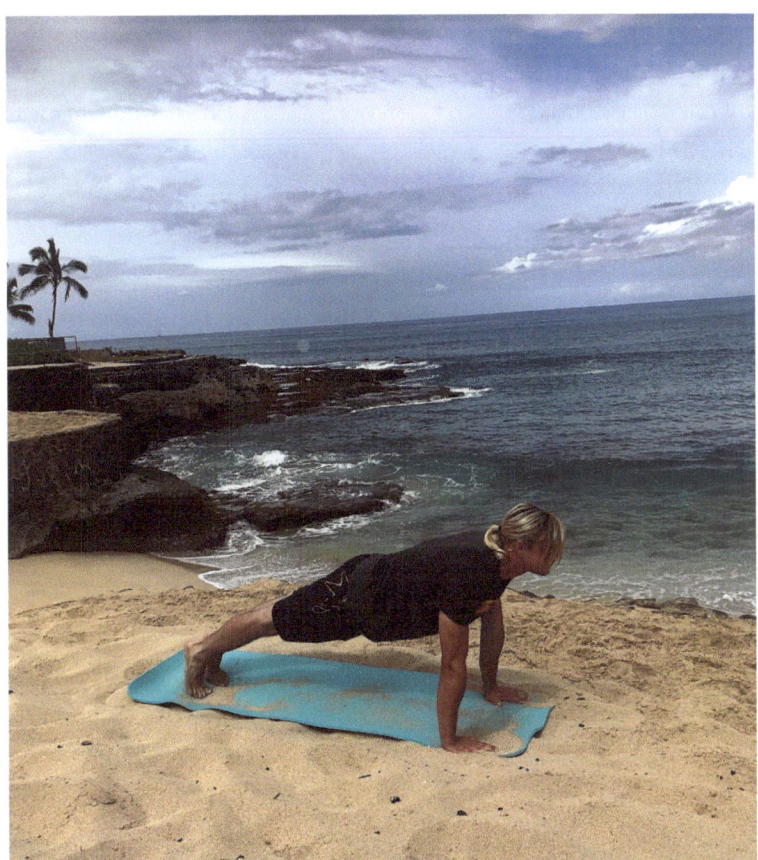

Try exploring your inner garden as we go through the next poses. Look around within you. What else is there? Discover the inner garden as if you were taking a relaxing walk in a beautiful nature preserve. As you move your body and hold the image of the garden, you are fine tuning your *on-the-go* meditation skills.

Slowly drop down onto the mat. Relax your feet and legs. Let your toes take a rest on the mat while moving into **Cobra** pose. Shift the work of this pose to your stomach, shoulders, back, chest and arms. Keep your elbows bent.

Feel the strength of your force field under you. See yourself in your inner garden and hold this pose until both arms are exhausted. Curl your toes back under to come up into **Downward Dog** or **Ardo Muhka Savasana.**

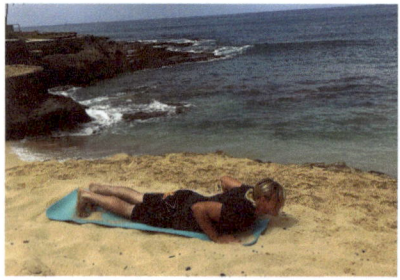 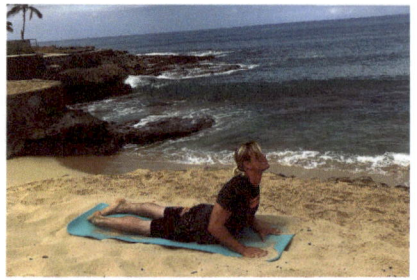

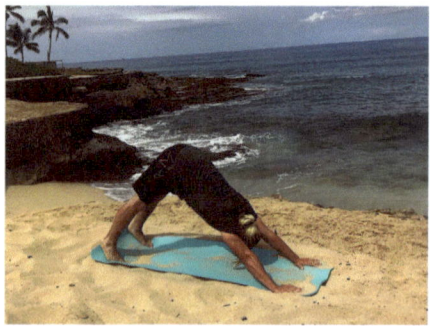

There are several key points to getting the most out of **Downward Dog.** Learn to use your feet and hands as stabilizers. Push the palms of your hands firmly into the mat, spread out all of your fingers and then place the fingers down and grip with them. Your fingers and toes should act more like suction cups that geckos have for climbing a wall.

Push your heels back to take some of the weight off your toes. Both hips should be even. Check to make sure your back is flat. Hold this pose until your arms are tired. Bring one foot up beside your hands and then the other, returning to the front of the mat.

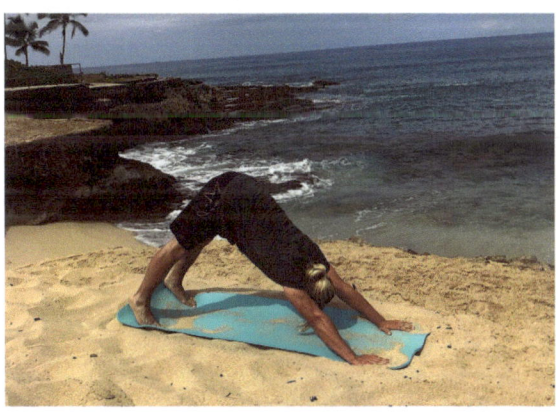

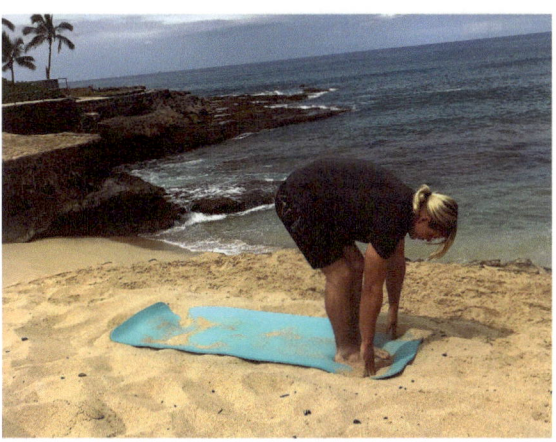

Sit back into **Chair** pose and reach both arms out in front of you. Extend both arms up as you push into **Tadasana.** Breathe the Ha deeply for a few breaths. Prepare to repeat this sequence leading with the right foot moving back.

The sequence is **Tadasana, Forward Bend, Extended Forward Bend, Runner's Lunge, Plank** pose, **Cobra, Downward Dog, Chair** pose and back to **Tadasana**. Always do both sides. Use all the skills you have learned: scapulae flat, Ha breathing, Fluidity, Ahimsa, and *on-the-go* meditation of *Mana Gardening*.

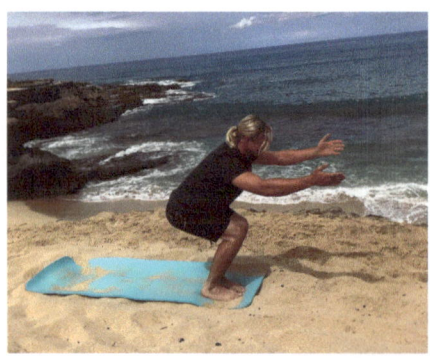
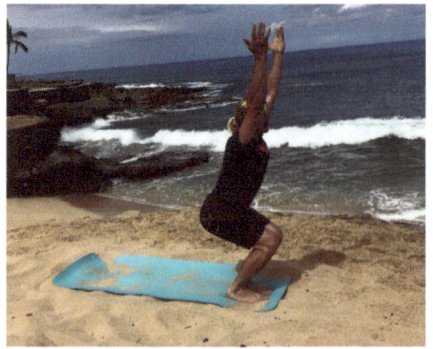

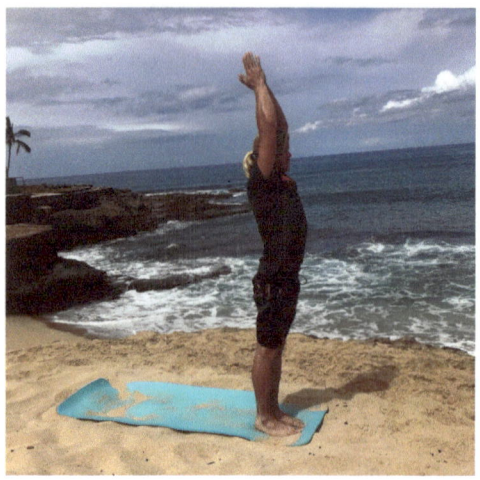

Celebrating the Mana

Complete your sun salutations on both sides and come into **Tree** pose or **Vriksasana** starting with your right foot up. Say, "Aloha" and celebrate the *Mana* growing stronger within you. You have built a force field to protect you from negativity. You are learning how to use *Mana Gardening on-the-go* meditation to access your inner energy anytime you want to feel relaxed or empowered.

Step back down into **Tadasana** and breathe. Come back into **Tree** pose with your left foot up. Breathe deeply and each time you exhale slowly say, "Ha." Embrace the power around you and within you.

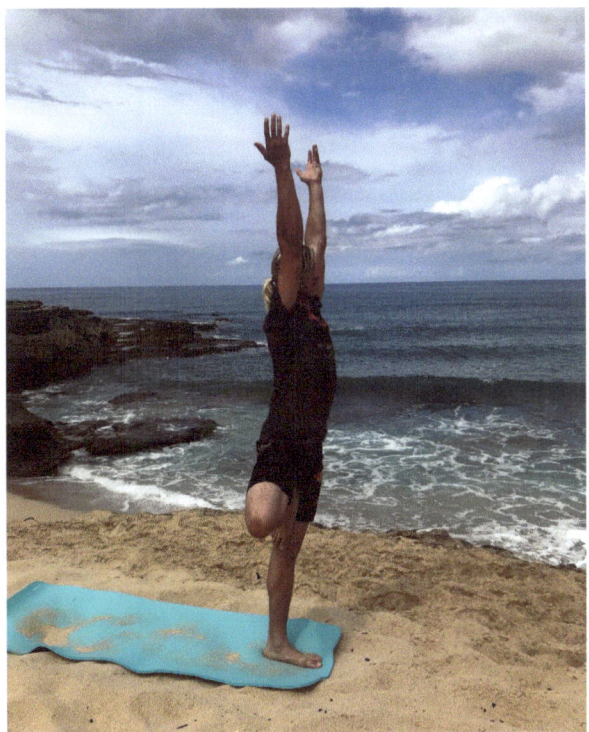

Come into a **Forward Bend** holding onto your ankles. Drop back into your inner garden and see yourself there relaxing as your upper body hangs here taking a few breaths. Your upper body should rise away from your legs as you inhale and sink close to your legs as you exhale.

Next place your right hand under your right toes and your left hand under your left toes. There will be a slight stretch to your legs, back and arms with this pose. Relax a few more breaths and enjoy this restorative pose.

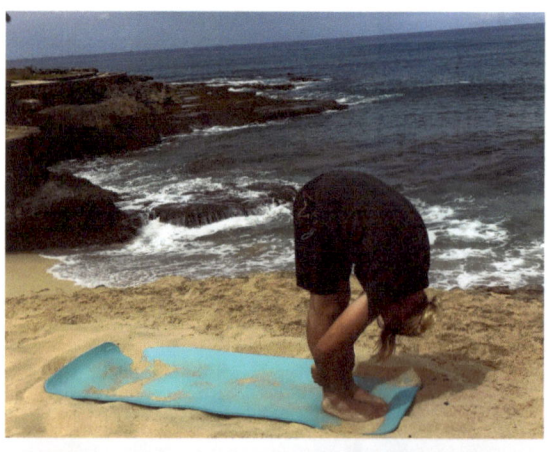

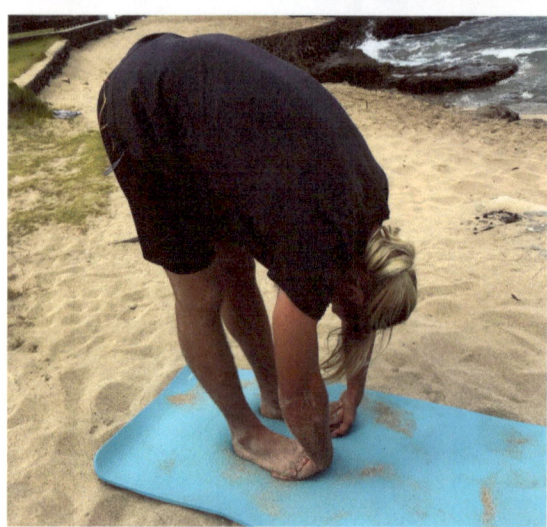

Come down onto the mat and come into **Hero** pose. If needed, sit on a block or folded blanket. Make sure that you are practicing good posture. See yourself in your inner garden relaxing. Exhale the Ha slowly for three fully focused, deep breaths.

Lean forward with both arms outstretched for **Balasana**, or **Child's** pose. With proper alignment, this simple, restorative pose offers extraordinary benefits. The next two pages discuss the secrets to achieving the most from **Balasana.**

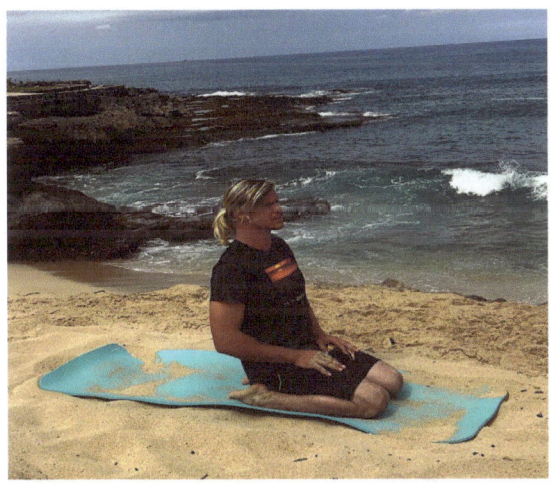

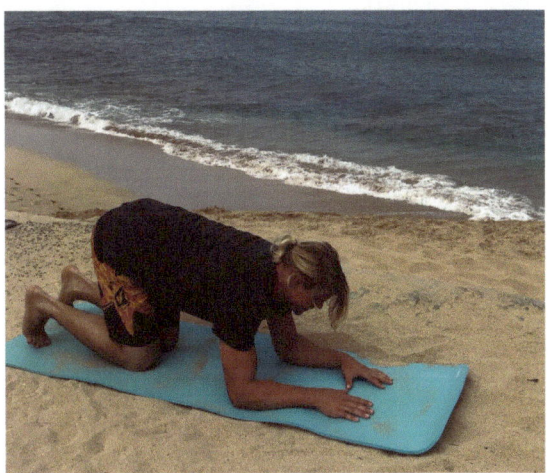

The Secrets of Balasana

Balasana or **Child's** pose holds many secrets. This pose should be called the fountain of youth pose. It has the power to keep us fluid, and it has the power to heal. Invest some time learning how to get the most of this pose.

Start from **Hero** pose, and make sure your knees are hip-distance apart. Use a block or blanket to sit on if you feel any strain in your back, hips or knees. Be sure you do not have any impingements and be sure you have proper posture.

Lean forward with both arms stretched out in front of your body. Try using a block under your head at first. Slowly relax your head, neck, shoulders and arms. Submit to gravity and feel the grounding power of the earth. This pose rewards, and decompresses every part of the spine.

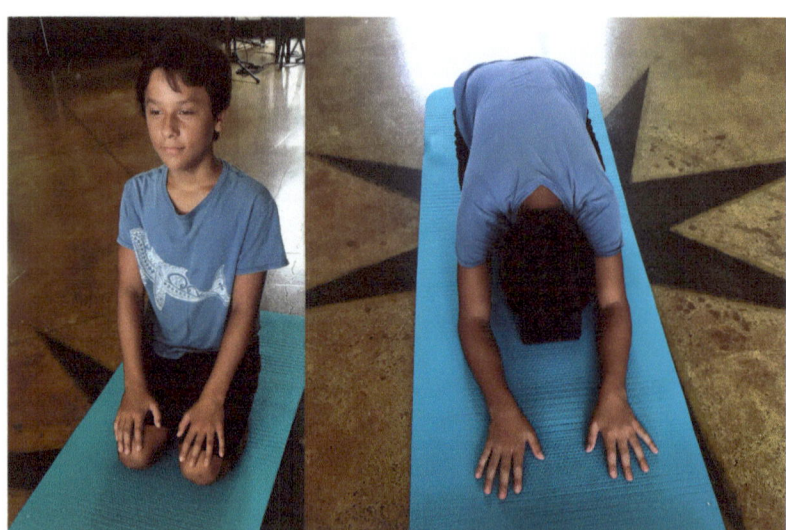

Experiment with optional ways to do **Balasana.** Try removing the block and resting your head on the mat. Elongate the spine, move your arms to the side and let them rest beside your torso. Ask yourself what feels the most comfortable. Once you know how to fully relax in this pose, sink into this pose and let the weight of the world leave your body.

One of the secrets to this pose is that you can do it whenever you need to release stress–you can do it in bed before you go to sleep, or you can do this pose when you don't have time for a full yoga practice. This pose restores and rejuvenates your body with no effort other than gravity. Make this your go-to pose to release worries, drama or negative energy. Let the stress flow out from you and visualize your inner garden. See yourself there resting like a child and feel young again.

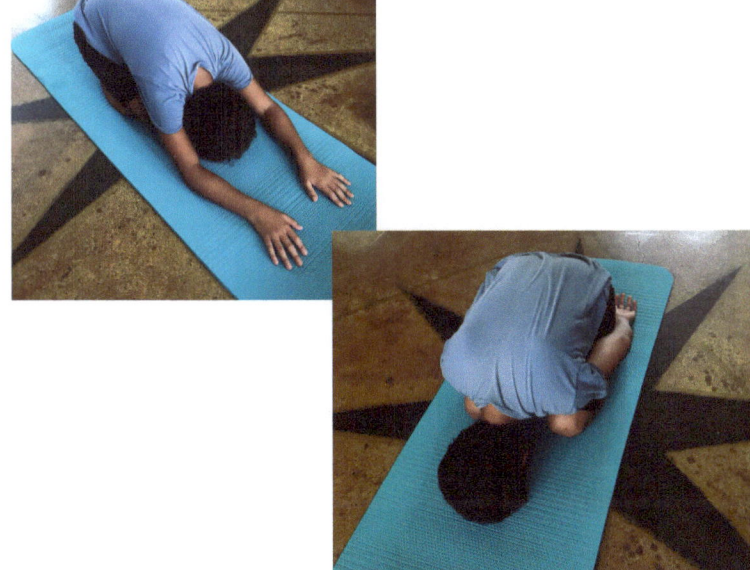

Sit up straight extending both legs forward into **Dandasana.** Tighten your stomach and leg muscles and then relax your muscles. Reflect in silence on what you have learned. You have corrected your posture and created a positive energy force field to safeguard you from negativity. You have visualized an inner paradise, your own idea of heaven and placed yourself there to relax and become empowered.

You have discovered that you can meditate while fluidly moving through a focused yoga practice. You are beginning to understand Ahimsa and how to move away from pain or impingements. You now use the Hawaiian Ha and see the importance of exhaling fully. Embrace the power of all your accomplishments and prepare to discover your inner *Mana* through a deeper **Suvasana**.

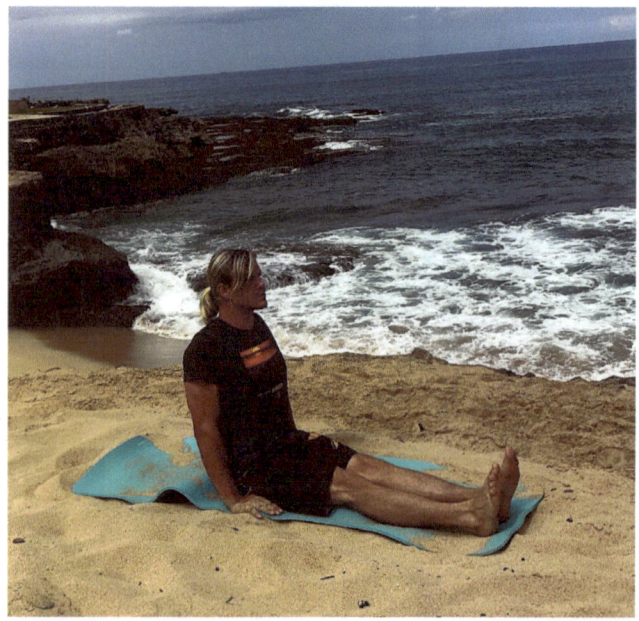

Sacred Suvasana

We believe that **Suvasana** is sacred. It allows the physiological sympathetic nervous system with all its energy from movement to embrace the parasympathetic nervous system in a moment of complete and total peace. Never, ever skip **Suvasana**. In this pose your conscious and subconscious processes can flow together freely bringing you great *Mana*.

Take a Pohaku Naholoholo traveling stone into the palm of each hand. Lay down onto the mat and be sure you have flat scapulae, a natural curve of spine, with relaxed legs and arms. Imagine a forthright energy flowing within you like a river filling a beautiful lake. This river is the energy of the universe and the lake is your *Mana*. See yourself walk to the edge of the lake and dip each stone into your *Mana*. See yourself wade into the water and relax floating in your inner power. Take five minutes of silence there.

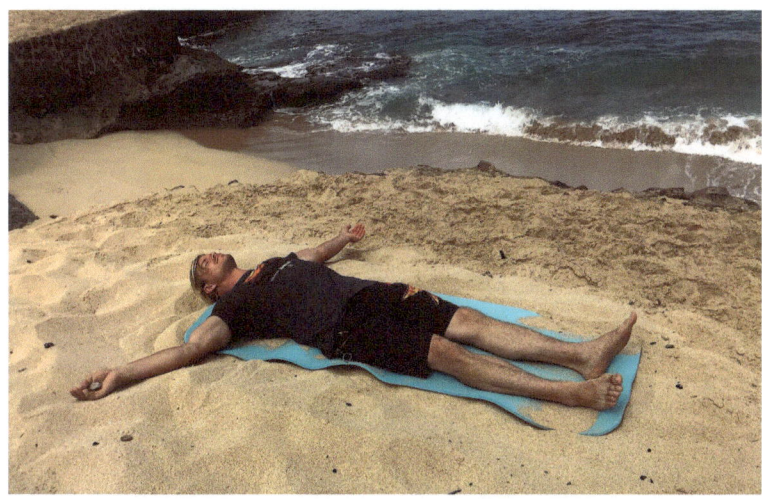

The Power of Mana

Aloha and welcome back. You have now filled these stones with *Mana* from within. This stored energy can be recycled whenever you feel tired or stressed. You may retrieve the positive energy you have stored in the stones or give these stones to someone you love when they need your strength.

These stones should remind you of that moment in time when you were deep within yourself and at total peace with everything in the universe. Place your stones somewhere you can glance upon them from time to time. When you see or touch them remember how truly empowered you are. Within you is an endless waterfall of energy that has the power to rejuvenate or relax you.

Your *Mana* is a private reserve of empowering energy, there to give you whatever you need whenever you need it. You can do this practice with beads or even pennies, as the Hawaiians believe everything has the ability to store and return the forthright energy of *Mana*.

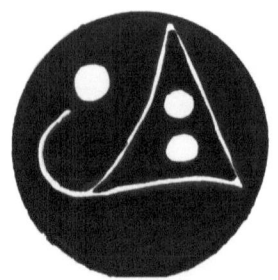

Your Mana Sciences Yogi

Your guide through this *Empower Me Free Yoga* flow is a Registered Yoga Teacher (RYT), trained in Hatha yoga and is certified in Mana Sciences Hawaiian Empowerment Techniques for Yoga. Known as "Cosmo", he offers private classes on the island of Oahu and specializes in yoga for those who want to retain their mobility. He credits yoga as the key to his recovery after a major injury. You can find out more about Cosmo at www.cosmouniversalyoga.com or his site registered with Yoga Alliance under Cosmo Universal Yoga at www.yogaalliance.org

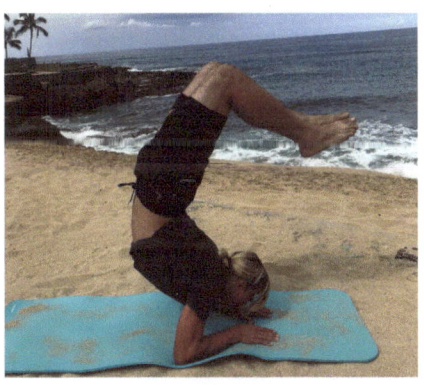

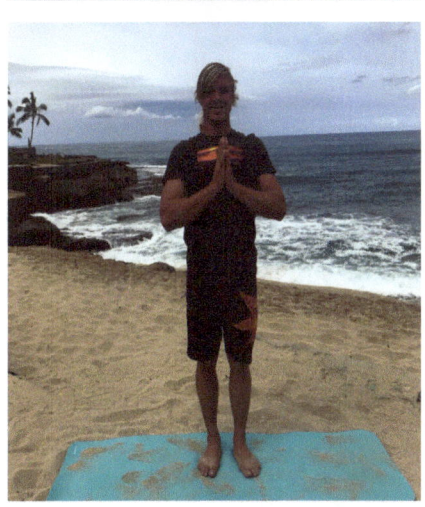

Keti Kamalani and Michelle Shine, Ph.D. are dedicated to sharing the ancient Hawaiian wisdom of *Mana Gardening*. They now offer the opportunity for Registered Yoga Teachers to become certified in Mana Sciences Hawaiian Empowerment Techniques for Yoga.

Mana Gardening Institute, LLC is a woman-owned, Hawaii-based organization established to facilitate scientific research in forthright personal empowerment and *Mana Gardening* techniques. Visit the website to learn more about Mana Sciences and Mana Psychology research and follow us on Facebook/Twitter/Instagram under ManaGardening.

www.managardening.com

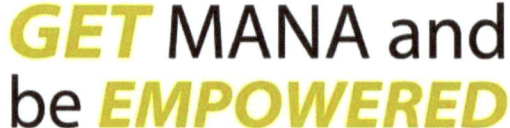

www.ingramcontent.com/pod-product-compliance
Lightning Source LLC
Chambersburg PA
CBHW040315010626

45792CB00022B/336